HELP ME, LORD — I HURT

HELP ME, LORD — I HURT

Virgina Thompson

Harvest House Publishers
Irvine, California 92714

HELP ME, LORD—I HURT

Copyright © 1978 Harvest House Publishers
Irvine, California 92714
Library of Congress Catalog Card Number 78-55505
ISBN 0-89081-145-8

Printed in the United States of America.

To my father, Harold Volk,
whose faith has kept him strong
through all of life's hurts.

CONTENTS

I. **When It's God and Me** 11
This Special Moment 13
You Know Me 15
Loneliness 17
Simply Trust 19
Turmoil 21
Surgery 23
Psalm Of Love 25
Time Out 27
Inadequate 29
He Answers Me 31
Where Is Your God? 33
Added Hours 35
Self-Discipline 37
Time 39
Confusion 41
Thanksgiving 43

II. **On The Home Front** 45
He Expects The Best 47
My Security 49
Monday Nights 51
Moods 53
Defensive 55
More Than Words 57
Doubt Bucket 59
Not Totally Understood 61
Just For Us 63
Help My Budget 65

Us 67
Nature Heals 69
Sunday Morning 71
Guilt 73
Not Yet Finished 75
Remember The Meadow 77
Hurts 79
Death's Blow 81
Your Promises Are True 83

III. **What Others See** 85
Smile 87
Honesty Hurts 89
Seeking Forgiveness 91
Too Committed 93
Avoidance 95
Harsh Words 97
I Hate Good-Byes 99
Envy 101
I Care 103
Insecure 105
The Gift of Friendship 107
Make Me Willing 109
You and I, Lord 111

HELP ME, LORD –
I HURT

I

When It's God And Me

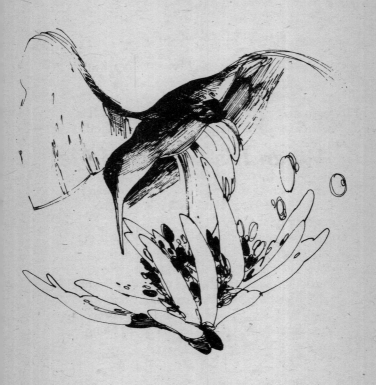

THIS SPECIAL MOMENT

Lord, I am jumping inside. Good things are all
around me. I am surrounded with blessings
and honors. I enjoy health of mind, body,
and spirit. I cherish this special moment. It is
mine to live and to savor each minute detail.
My direction is clear. My motives are above
reproach. I view my troubled world from
above. There is hope running through my
veins. I can't remember yesterday, nor can I
think of tomorrow. But I soak in the rays of
your sunlight today.
This moment I will always remember. I will
call it back when tribulation knocks at my
door. I will use it as a stepping stone when
my body is weary at the end of my day. I will
tell others of the satisfaction of knowing you.
Thank you, Lord, for drawing near to me, for
showing me that you love me, and for being
my special friend.

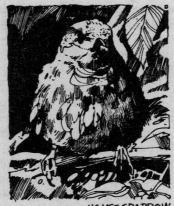

HOUSE SPARROW

YOU KNOW ME

Lord, I so often tell you about my needs, my desires, my wants, and my ambitions. Oftentimes I even list them for you so that you will understand exactly what it is that I am trying to convey. I remind you of how faithful I have been. I make sure that I include my weariness, my overwhelming responsibilities, and the exhausting demands on me. I want you to comprehend each detail.

Somehow this morning, I am reminded that you notice every sparrow that falls to the ground. You have even numbered the hairs on my head. Why, you most certainly are aware of my needs. You are a God of infinite detail. Detail that I cannot even comprehend.

Perhaps, Lord, the lists are important for my finite mind. Perhaps they are necessary for my understanding, but you certainly do not need them. Not one thought of mine goes unnoticed or unheeded by you. As I think of the complexity of my being and simplicity with which you lead me, it seems a paradox.

Teach me to see the beauty and to know the meaning of simple trust . . . of simple faith. Help me remember that as long as you have my total will committed to you, you will provide for each of my needs. You will heed every desire and you will control all of my ambitions.

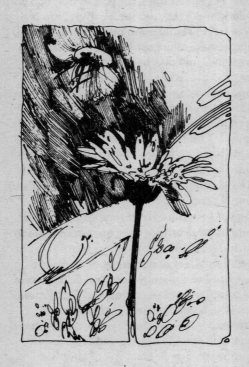

LONELINESS

Loneliness hovers over me this evening. There is an emptiness way down deep within. In a way, I am frightened as if a storm was brewing and I needed shelter. It really hurts for a few moments and then subsides to a dull ache. I cannot tie the feeling to any conscience awareness. I am just plain lonely.

Dear Lord, I draw near to you for comfort and for protection. I ask that you make your presence felt. Show me that you are near and you do really care.

If only the phone would ring, and someone would say "I care." Often you use people to show us your love.

While I wait, is there someone else who is lonely that you want me to phone? Someone who is experiencing hurt or disappointment? Do you have a job for me to do? Will my loneliness subside when I reach out my hand to someone else?

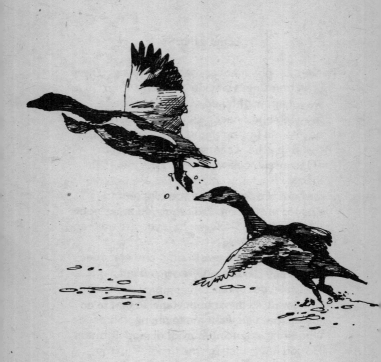

SIMPLY TRUST

Hear my voice, Oh Lord; guide me with your
   hand.
   Today begins my new adventure with you.
   I wait for your instructions.
   I wait patiently for you to show me what to
   do.
And I hear you answer,
   "Begin each day listening for the creative
      ways that I wish for you to follow."
   "Begin to live in a constant attitude of
      prayer."
   "I will teach you."
   "I will encourage you."
   "I will set you upright when you fall."
   "I will be your constant companion."
   "Trust me. It is not important for you to do
      the work; you need not even try."
   "Simply trust me. Leave all to me."

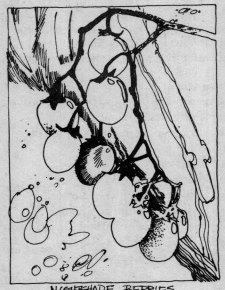

NIGHTSHADE BERRIES

TURMOIL

O God, my God, this turmoil inside of me—
 the turmoil of the every day nitty-gritty cares
 and pressures—is getting close to destroying
 me.
 Come near me with your acceptance and
 your love.
 Surround me as I meditate on your Word.
 Hold the enemy back and don't let his
 attacks of discouragement cause me to
 falter.
I thank you for all of the times that you have
 given me peace in the midst of turmoil.
 I praise your name for allowing me to
 experience these feelings so that I can better
 realize that I am nothing without you.
 You are the only one who can turn the
 tempest into calm.
 You are the only one who can assure me that
 I need to relax and to let go.
 You will take care of the problems that cause
 me turmoil.

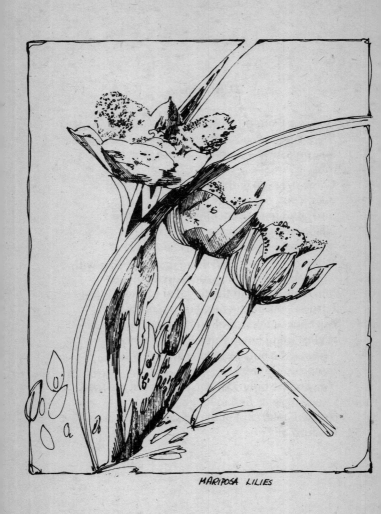

MARIPOSA LILIES

SURGERY

Draw near to me, Lord. So many uncertainties
  are flooding my mind. I have never faced
  surgery before.
What if—there is a malignancy?
  Who will care for my little ones?
  I am still young.
  I'm not ready for weighty decisions.
  I'm not yet prepared.
  I must find peace.
  Don't hide your face from me, but come with
  your strength to replace my weakness.
I am crying for the comfort that you promised.
  I am praying for confidence and peace.
You know me better than I know myself.
  You created me. You bought me. You
  planned every day of my life. Assure me
  once more. Show me that you have control
  now and that nothing can separate me from
  your love.
Thank you, Lord. I trust. I believe.

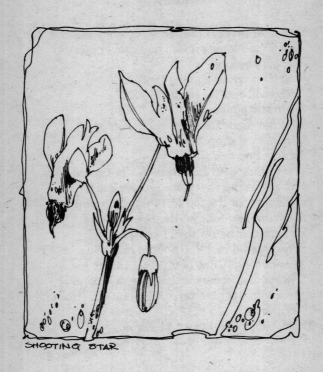

SHOOTING STAR

PSALM OF LOVE

Lord, I write my psalm of love to you this day.
  You are above all else to me.
  I choose to carry my cross for you.
  I thank you for the lessons I've learned.
I thank you for holding my hand through four
  surgeries.
  It is because of you that my doctor said,
  "I can't believe it. You 'go out' smiling and
  'come to' smiling."
  It is because you have always been with me.
I thank you for sitting with me week after week,
  while I waited my turn for the routine blood
  tests.
  I became accustomed to the familiar
  medicine smell;
  I enjoyed acquaintances with the lab
  assistants.
  You always prepared me for the outcome.
  "Sorry, take your medicine . . . your two
  shots . . . and we'll see you again next
  week."
For nearly ten years, you taught me needed
  lessons through physical suffering. Your
  lessons seemed harsh at times. But I thank
  you for them all.
Best of all, I thank you for a doctor who cares
  for me especially—who did all that he knew
  how—before referring me to another. And I
  thank you for the wisdom of medicine
  through which I received a workable answer
  to my body's rebellion.

You speak to me.

"It appears that mentally, emotionally, and spiritually you handle life very well. But your physical body can only tolerate a certain amount of stress. When it reaches that level, your blood chemistry becomes imbalanced. I prescribe two to three days a month away from your normal demands, preferably alone."

And Lord of mine, I am a new person.

When I go away, I return physically ready to keep up with my other selves—my mind, my emotions and my spirit.

I guess that's why you "went away" when you were here on earth.

Thank you for the example.

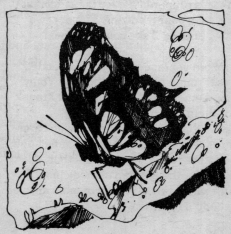

TIME OUT

Lord, my cold has me feeling low today.
    The chill of winter has a depressing affect
    upon my being.
    Food lures its ugly temptations before me.
    "Here, eat away the blahs," it calls.
Complex and busy are my days, with little time
    for the simple, the important things.
    I long to pray, to meditate, to bask in your
    presence.
    I desire to know neatness and order in my
    day.
    The claws of clutter are tearing at me hourly.
Have mercy on me, renew my spirit.
    Protect me from the trivia roundabout me.
    There are those who would cause my
    conservation to be shallow and void of
    purpose.
    May the words I speak have meaning and be
    preceded with thoughts of you.
Lord, I have set aside this day to retreat and to
    renew. As I turn my thoughts towards you,
    fill me with freshness of mind, of soul, and of
    spirit.
I feel your calm. I sense a quieting in my spirit.
    Guide me this day as you do the planets in
    the heavens. May the timing of my activities
    be as perfect as their steady obedience to the
    orbit that you have charted for them.

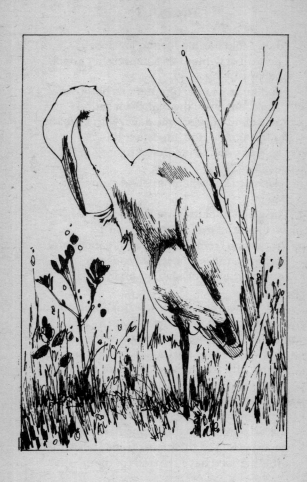

INADEQUATE

Lord, all day I have been fighting a sense of
 inadequacy.
 Can I go into my social world tonight and
 interact with confidence and poise?
I'm trusting in you, my God.
 Prepare me.
 Show me what it is that you would have me
 wear.
 Pick out the garment in which I can best
 represent you.
 Guide my hand as I comb every hair into
 place and as I apply my makeup.
I will hold my head high and my shoulders
 straight for you will restore my confidence
 and set me on my feet once more.
I will walk into my evening trusting in your
 invisible support.
 I am mindful of your continual presence in
 my life.
 May I reflect you to others.

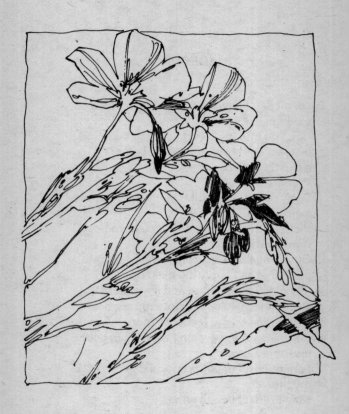

HE ANSWERS ME

I feel inadequate . . .
  "Ye are the salt of the earth."
I feel lonely . . .
  "I will never leave you nor forsake you."
I feel put upon . . .
  "I was crucified."
I feel overwhelmed . . .
  "You can do all things through Christ who
  strengthens you."

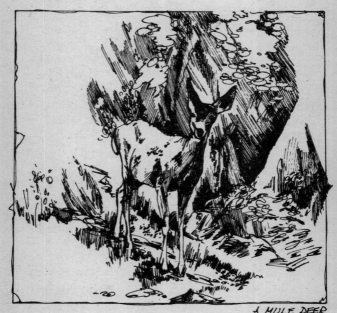

A MULE DEER

WHERE IS YOUR GOD?

Lord, I am sick inside. I am helpless. Hope is
   not in sight.
   If you don't come and rescue me, I am sure
   to be destroyed.
   My enemies are laughing at my predicament
   because I trusted in you in the first place.
   They say to me,
      "Where is your God now?"
      "Why doesn't He rescue you from this
      pit?"
      "He will let you die here."
Lord, show your face and reveal your power so
   that everyone will know that I was right
   when I trusted you.
   I have followed you right up to this very
   moment and I believe that you have charted
   my entire way of hope and faith.
   I give you every detail of my day.
   I choose to trust you right now . . . for
   direction for the next 15 minutes . . . that is
   as long as I can handle right now.
   I need moment-by-moment direction.

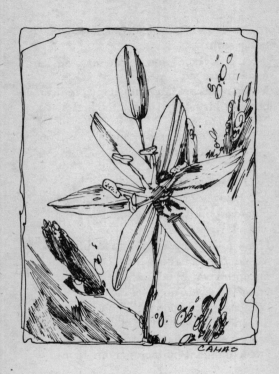

CAMAD

ADDED HOURS

I praise you Lord.
   This very day you have given me your peace.
   Early this morning I turned my busy
   schedule over to you and you have surely
   added hours to my day.
   You have increased my efficiency a
   hundredfold. You have even provided
   moments to meditate and to rest.
   You caused unnecessary responsibilities to
   vanish before me. You directed my path
   towards the positive and the urgent duties.
Thank you, Lord, for showing me your mercy
   and your loving-kindness. Thank you for
   showering my day with pleasant thought and
   with laughter. How mindful you are of my
   needs. I will bless your name all the days of
   my life. I will share your tender mercies with
   those around me.

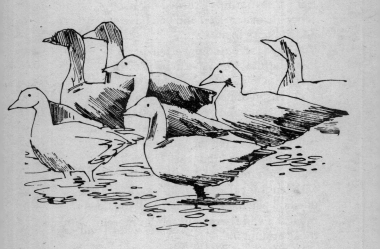

SELF-DISCIPLINE

Lord, I am engaged in an inner conflict.
Thank you for being my personal God.
This conflict will destroy me if you do not
rescue me with your strength.

On one hand, I desire to be self-indulgent for
brief moments of pleasure. But I am aware
that if I discipline myself, I can reap a
harvest of long range fulfillment.

Strengthen me. Help me see beyond my
immediate desire and catch a glimpse of the
person that you want to make of me.

My resistance is low and my enemies see me as
a sure catch for their trap. Deliver me out of
my conflict and set my feet firmly upon a
solid decision.

I will praise your name forever and ever. I will
sing your praises evermore.

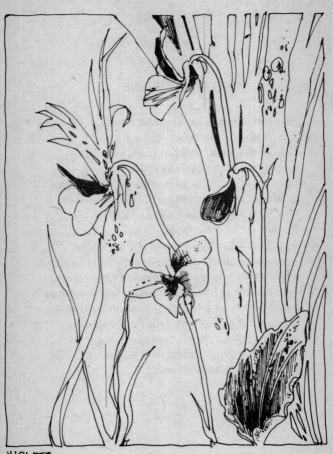

VIOLETS

38

TIME

Time is of no real importance to you as long as
   you have my will, Lord.
   Today is half gone and the evil one threatens
   that I'd better get to work or I'll be meeting
   failure when the sun sets. He accuses me of
   possessing no real value.
   The sun is overhead and here I sit . . . gazing
   at the fire . . . listening to the wind outside . .
   enjoying your presence.
Draw near to me as those who accuse me flee
   from your presence. You have a plan for my
   day. As you call me into action, may I readily
   respond. Thank you for providing me a rest
   stop and a time of reflection. Give me the
   ability to relax. Thank you for today.

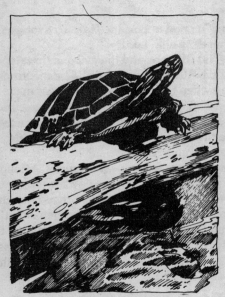

AN EASTERN PAINTED TURTLE

CONFUSION

Lord, you have promised to be my guide . . .
  to give me direction,
  but the enemy of confusion surrounds my
  day.
  I see so many immediate demands on my
  time.
  This confusion hinders all of my progress.
  When I start in one direction of
  responsibility,
  I am accused that I am neglecting greater
  areas of need.
Oh hear my plea for help. Give me the wisdom
  to sort out my priorities and then to measure
  my time accordingly.
  Put me inside a bubble of your love.
  Don't let confusion penetrate close enough
  to do harm.
I remember the many times you have directed
  my day to perfection, and I pray that you'll
  do so now. I do not ask you to clear all of the
  difficult situations from my path. I only ask
  that you gently guide me either around them
  or through them.
  I must be certain of you guidance.
  When the enemy accuses me, I'll stand
  strong in the knowledge that I followed your
  direction.
Thank you, Lord, for the assurance that you are
  in charge.
  You are directing my steps.

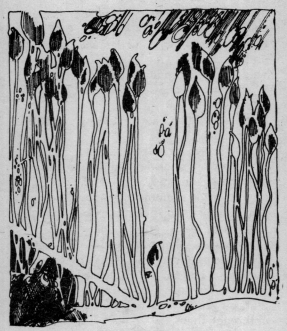

POLYTRICHUM MOSS SPORE PODS

THANKSGIVING

In the midst of misunderstanding, I lift my
    voice in praise and thanksgiving to you,
    Lord. You are truly a Holy God. You have
    promised me faith, hope and love.
Why, then should I be downhearted or cast
    down by my enemies? They can harm my
    body. They can damage my emotions. Yes,
    they can even take my life.
But God, control my soul. You control my will
    and my thoughts. No one can enter and snuff
    out my faith. It is steadfast. Neither can hope
    be stolen, nor the love that you have placed
    within me be robbed.
I relax in your peace. I have that blessed
    assurance that no misunderstanding can
    separate me from your love—my God and
    my Saviour.

II

On The Home Front

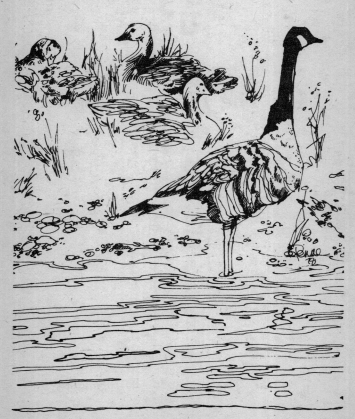

CANADIENNE GEESE / GOSLINGS

HE EXPECTS THE BEST

Lord, he has always expected the best from
  me.
  He has never let me be satisfied with a job
  half done.
  He has expected the best in how I look.
  He has expected the best in my attitude
  towards life.
  He has expected the best in my professional
  involvements.
  He has expected me to be the best wife.
  He has expected me to be the best mother.
  He has expected the best in my homemaking,
  cooking and entertaining.
Oftentimes I resented it.
  I wanted to be satisfied with good intentions.
  I struggled with his demands.
  I thought they were too hard.
But today I thank you, Lord.
  I thank you that his expectations have always
  been the highest for me.
  I thank you that he has had confidence in me.
  I am still striving.
  I haven't arrived.
  I am still struggling over his expectations of
  me.
  If he didn't always expect the best, I might

have become complacent and satisfied.
I would not be the woman I am today.
May I also expect the best of others.
May I not let them stop short of their life's
goals because I didn't expect enough of
them.

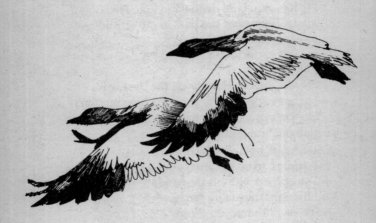

MY SECURITY

Lord, he is away tonight and I am left with the responsibility of the children and the house. I have a hollow spot inside of me. It's as if my security has been taken away. Usually at this time of night I am snuggled down with a good book and ready to fall asleep.

Tonight it is different. I was fine until the sun bid adieu. But the evening shadows robbed me of any desire to be alone.

I pray that you will come near to me. Allow me to feel your encompassing love and presence.

This void within me needs to be filled. Assure me that you are still in control and I need not depend on his presence. It is best when he is here. But you, my God, are my strength and my security.

Thank you. You have filled me with your peace.

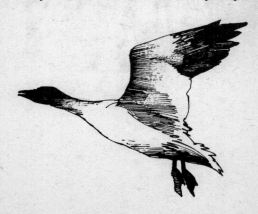

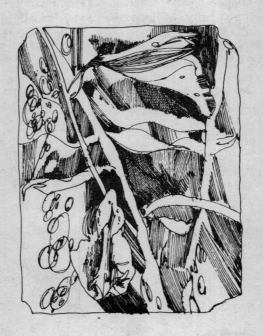

MONDAY NIGHTS

This is a beautiful summer evening, Lord. I'd
   like to take a ride, visit friends, or maybe
   take the children swimming. It is hard for me
   to understand the importance of ''Monday
   night baseball.'' I just can't get into it like
   the men folk.

And if I may complain a bit, Monday nights are
   awful the year around. Football in the fall,
   basketball in the winter, and baseball in the
   summer. Must I always give in to Monday
   nights?

I took a bike ride, and I pulled some weeds. I
   even baked a cake for tomorrow's lunches.
   There is nothing left to do.

Lord, you always show me how trite I am.
   Okay, I'll see what the score is, and give it
   another Monday night try.

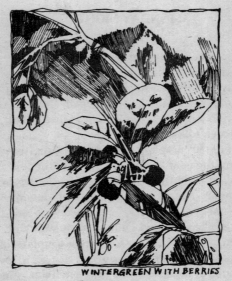

WINTERGREEN WITH BERRIES

MOODS

Lord, I don't understand how one minute I can
feel secure in his arms and the next minute
be enraged by his words.
This morning there was a beautiful bond
between us and for a change we weren't
even rushed. We were leisurely beginning
our day, Saturday. A new day. The world
was ours for the taking.
I can't remember his words.
To me they were accusing.
I know that he said them and then forgot it.
But I began to smolder inside, while my
outward reactions to him progressed from
cool to cold.
It is already afternoon and I still suffer inside.
It's crazy. He is watching the ball game
totally unaware of how I feel towards him.
Now I am hating myself — my childish self.
Cleanse me, Lord. Clean out the wound. Begin
my healing so that I can again be free to love.
Forgive me for overreacting and for wasting
this beautiful day.
I will be grateful to you all of my days. I will
come to you more quickly next time.
Thank you.

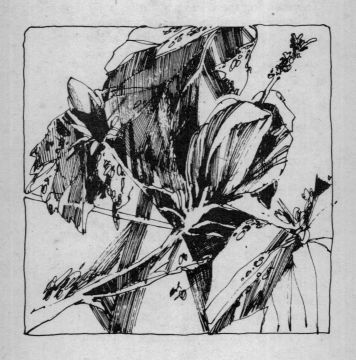

DEFENSIVE

I was certainly defensive, Lord. I didn't like
   being told that I had left the faucet dripping
   again. I guess to me it really wasn't that
   important. A dripping faucet just doesn't
   bother me.
Whether or not the faucet drips isn't the issue.
   The problem lies deep inside of me. I resent
   being told that I am wrong. I immediately
   get defensive and quickly justify my actions.
Lord, dig out the weeds of defensiveness from
   my personality. Set me free from their
   strangling runners. They have the power to
   destroy.
   Plant within me a free spirit, I pray, that will
   bring a new fragrance into my personality—
   a spirit that will take the threat out of being
   told that I am in error.
Thank you for again hearing my prayer.

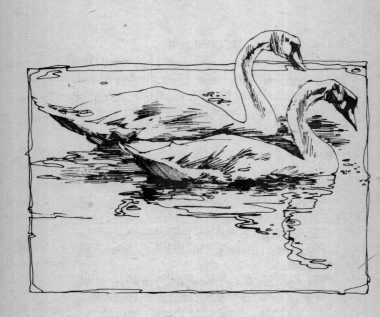

MORE THAN WORDS

He wanted to talk, Lord. I wanted to listen. But things didn't go well. I didn't respond the way he expected or needed. He put up a wall and now my words bounce back to me. They are not penetrating through his soundproof structure.

Please, Lord, I ask you to give me another try. Give me the wisdom to help him solve the uncertainty that he is facing. May I hear more than his mere words. May I tune in to his world. May I listen carefully and then encourage him to dream dreams . . . to set goals . . . and to develop plans to reach those goals.

I depend upon you, God. Without you, I'll fail him. Without you, he will fail to fulfill the plan you have for his life.

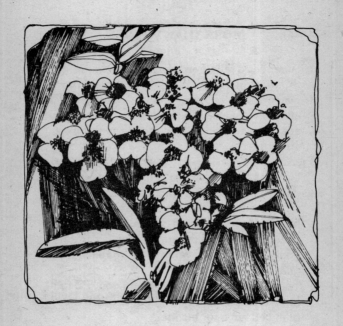

DOUBT BUCKET

Dear Lord,
   I am puzzled by his ability to unlock my
   "Doubt bucket."
   Just when I think I have secured all of my
   fears and doubts under the lid, locked it, and
   thrown away the key, he comes along and
   begins to pry on the lid or to pick the lock.
   Before I know it, the entire bucket explodes
   in my face.
He reminds me that I failed to find out what
   time our son will be in from his date. He
   questions why I would drive twenty miles
   without a spare tire. When I pull the cover
   under my chin at night, he asks if I locked
   the door and set the alarm.
O God, give me confidence in my decisions so
   that all of my doubts and fears will be locked
   up forever. I will be grateful to you and I will
   praise your name.

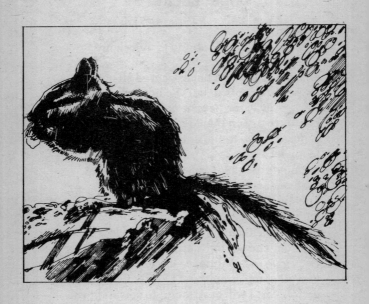

NOT TOTALLY UNDERSTOOD

Lord, I cannot totally understand him.
    I cannot understand his inner motives.
    I can only see and react to his actions.
Likewise, he cannot totally understand me.
    He cannot interpret all of my needs.
    He can only act upon his concept of them.
I feel that if we fully understand each other,
    we would not have to depend on you, our
    Creator. Because there is no human being
    able to comprehend my deepest hurts and
    joys, I must come to you freely and daily.
    You put every delicate part of my personality
    together and you know my every thought.
Forgive me for expecting him to go beyond the
    limits of his understanding of me. And
    forgive me for feeling defeat when I come to
    the ''no trespassing'' sign in his personality.
May I reverence the privacy that has been
    reserved for you and him to share; and may
    he never intrude upon the relationship that is
    uniquely yours and mine.

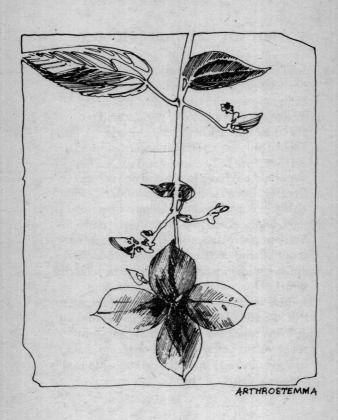

ARTHROSTEMMA

JUST FOR US

Lord, it was good to have my husband pop in
unexpectedly this afternoon. I thank you for
giving him to me. He is truly a man of
integrity. I am proud to be his wife and the
mother of his children.

You are aware of the many adjustments we
have both had to make. For several years it
seemed that we couldn't reach an agreement
on much of anything. But planted within
both of us was the desire and the willingness
to stick with it, no matter what.

You have honored our mutual desires to have a
loving, workable marriage which fulfills both
of our needs.

We are opposites in so many ways, Lord. Yet,
you have united our personalities to
accomplish a ministry designed just for us.

Thank you.

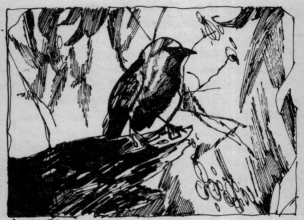

ALTAMIRA ORIOLE

HELP MY BUDGET

Lord, I am frustrated today over the ever
increasing cost of living. I have specific
needs today. Needs that are immediate . . .
Personal needs and family needs.

I am reminded of your words " . . . take no
thought of what ye shall eat or what ye shall
wear. My Father in heaven knoweth your
needs."

Free me from this doubt that harasses me. It
nags at me and destroys my ability to be free
and to create.

All of this world's riches are at your command.
You surely have a lesson for me. Perhaps I
cannot distinguish a need from a desire.
Teach me. May I never have so much that I
no longer consult you. It is when I am most
needy that I stay closest to you.

Provide me O God, with enough of this world's
goods that I won't become discouraged. But
keep me from having so much that I become
proud.

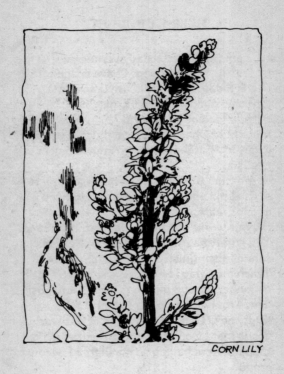

CORN LILY

US

Lord,*
>You have searched us and known us.
>You understand our every thought.
>You know when we lie down and when we
>get up.
>We cannot get away from your constant
>thoughts of us.
>Each of us was formed individually and in
>seclusion.

Now—we attempt to live as a whole—
>as a family unit.

It is amazing how you have brought our five
lives together into this home. We cannot
begin to understand one another, and each
of us becomes frustrated when we are not
understood.

I pray to you, God. I ask that you will take our
impatience, outspokenness, defensiveness,
selfish desires, and secret ambitions.

Melt each of us into a pliable consistency in
order that we can accept and respect the
complex personalities that make US—a
family.

*My paraphrase of Psalms 139

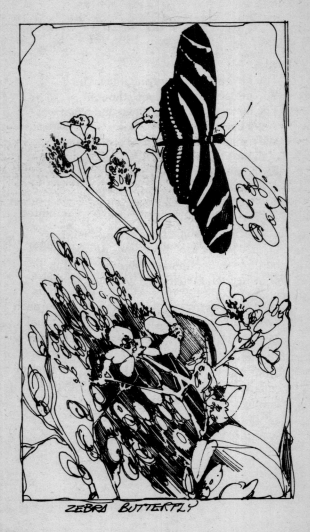

ZEBRA BUTTERFLY

NATURE HEALS

Lord, I pray that my family is having a
meaningful time. Perhaps the serenity of the
lake, the thrill of catching fish, and eating
fried chicken together will reduce the
tensions of togetherness that have mounted
during these past few weeks.
There have been foolish misunderstandings;
not horrendous grievances. Each has
trespassed and been trespassed against.
Unite them and soothe their relationships
with the silence of nature. May they see each
other as being unique, valuable, and equal.
You have various methods of healing broken
fellowship. I thank you for the confidence
that I have that you are at work in the lives of
my family. I thank you for the faith that I
have in you this day.

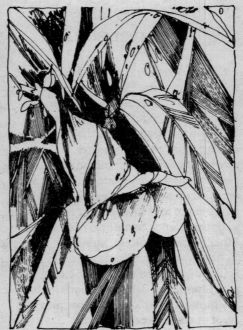

TRINITY PLANT

SUNDAY MORNING

Lord, I praise you while arising this Sunday
morning. It is good to prepare to go to your
house. How well I remember the confusion
that once reigned each and every Sunday.
Oh, how the enemy fought my efforts to have
harmony in our home. He caused us to sleep
in until there was a minimum of time.
Everyone was in someone else's way and
harsh words flew through the air as pointed
arrows, to cut and bruise the spirit of your
holy day. The bacon would burn. Clothes
weren't ready. The entire endeavor became
a calamity.

So I praise you this day—this Sunday—for the
way that you are defeating my enemies and
making Sunday morning a happy and
blessed time.

Your mercies to me are everlasting. They
endure forever.

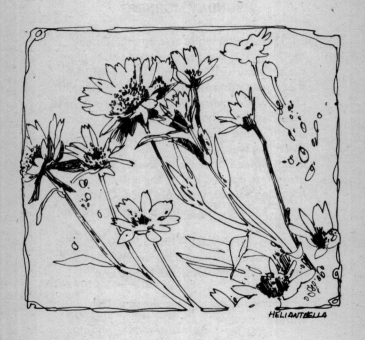

HELIANTHELLA

GUILT

Listen to me, Lord. Guilt has begun an ugly attack upon me. I made my decision. He would ride his bike to his ball game. He left unhappy. It is seven miles and he must ride in the traffic.

One side of me reasons that he needs to develop his independence as a fourteen-year-old. I also remember that I have needful limits on my time and my strength. But another part of me nags that I have sent him out into the five o'clock traffic. Will the long ride exhaust him before he begins his game?

Free me of this threatening guilt. It saps my strength and stalls all my creativity. In you, I've put my trust. I seek your guidance hourly. Judge my motives and honor me with your peace.

Protect him with your angels. Place a song within his heart. Let your understanding bind us together evermore.

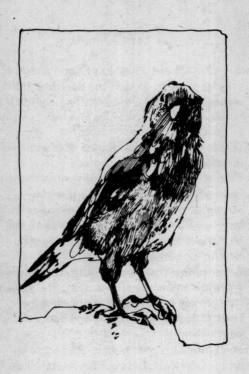

NOT YET FINISHED

Lord, when I drove up, he shut off the mower.
His manner was gentle as he picked up the
grey bundle from the porch and brought it to
me.
"What is it, Son?" I asked.
"A bird. He flew into the window. His neck
is broken."
The moment was a reverent one. Our spirits
were united while our thoughts were
individual and private.
It seems that too often his fourteen-year-old
ways are difficult for me to understand:
teasing his sister, cluttering up his room,
putting off his homework, and always having
the final word.
Grant to me the wisdom to see beyond his
turbulence and get a glimpse of the
gentleman that you are making.

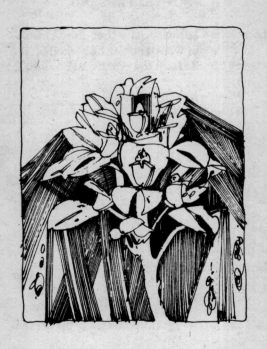

REMEMBER THE MEADOW

Lord, will he remember the meadow? He was
just a lad that hot summer afternoon when
we walked hand-in-hand along the mountain
path. Will he remember the bird that flew
along at our side, the ant that we stopped to
watch, and the bridge that we stood on as we
observed the clear water trickling over the
rocks?

He dropped my hand while we passed the
teenagers who were making merry on the
beach. What lad wants to be seen holding his
mother's hand?

Remember how we ran? How we laughed? And
how suddenly we stopped on that curve? It
was breathtaking—a meadow in the middle
of nowhere. We saw it at the same instant,
and we were both silenced by its beauty.

His hand slipped into mine again and we
bowed our heads in prayer.

"Thank you God, for a beautiful meadow."

Our steps back down the path were slow. Our
thoughts kept secret. We were united in
reverence, yet experiencing in solitude.

And remember what he said after we passed
those same teenagers?

"Mom, they don't even know about the
meadow."

We talked about life that day and agreed that

in the midst of the hassle there will always
be a meadow if we walk on.

He is a teenager now. Will he remember to
go on up the path and be renewed by the
serenity of the meadow?

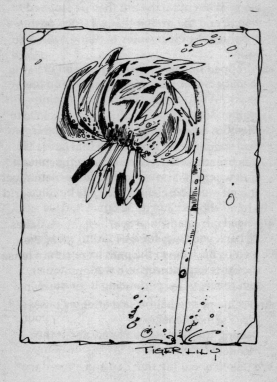

TIGER LILY

HURTS

It seems that everyone hurts. All people hurt in
some part of their life. I suppose that as long
as there is sin, there will be hurts.
Lord, give me strength today. Place within
me the ability to cast my hurt onto you. You
have already borne all of the hurt. You bore
it on Calvary. You have fought the sin battle
and you won the victory. Because of Calvary,
this victory is mine . . . Now . . . Today.
Have mercy and show your pardon and love to
my child this day. Release him from the
temptations that could destroy him. He is
your boy. I want to remind you that I gave
him to you. All rights to his life are yours, yet
distractions are calling to him from the world
around him.
Forgive me my sins and overlook my mistakes.
Bring to me your comfort. Relax all of the
parts of my mind and emotions that are tense
and burdened down with this great hurt.
Lord, as I trust you this moment for my own
peace and assurance, I also trust you to care
for his needs. I believe. I am singing your
praises for the mighty work that you are
about to perform in the life of one of my
children.

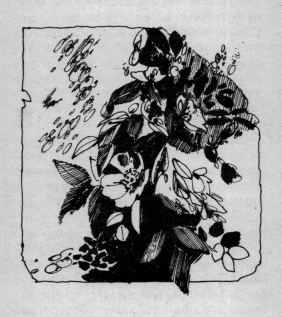

DEATH'S BLOW

My soul sings a song of Thanksgiving, O Lord.
You have heard my cry. You have honored
my request. You have quieted my fears and
my apprehensions.

As I lay on my bed wide-eyed, through the last
two nights, I was very much aware of the
battle that was raging between you and the
evil one. The bids were going higher for his
soul. You assured me during those hours
that the battle was yours to fight. You only
asked me to stay awake, to believe, and to be
calm.

Midway through the third night, the call came.
My only brother had slipped into eternity.
Amazing strength and peace held me during
the hours of informing the family and
making the necessary arrangements.

It appears to others to be such a tragedy, but
I stood by while the final blows were being
thrown.
You won, Lord. You won the battle.
I believe that you won in those final
moments.

It took three nights—a seeming parallel to your
death.
You asked me to watch and to pray.
I thank you for the privilege of sharing those
moments with you, and for preparing me for
his death.

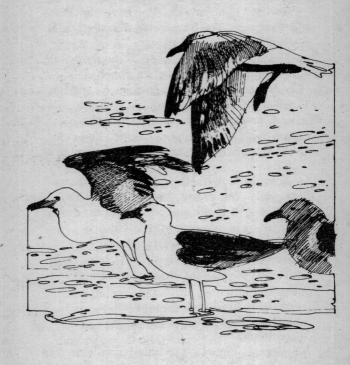

YOUR PROMISES ARE TRUE

Lord, it is well into the night, but sleep evades me. There is a sense of urgency deep within my spirit—an undefinable realization that you, my God, are at work. A battle is being fought.

My memory takes me back to the day I stood beside that mountain river. You whispered to me that just as the water was thrashing and twisting its way down the canyon—tugging at everything in its path—the day would come when my children would be out in the river of life, about to be destroyed by the evil thrusts of Satan.

You didn't stop there. You left me with the promise. I need only stand on the bank of life's river and support with my prayers. You will bring them to safety on the far shore.

I guess that's where I am—standing on the river bank. The only support I seem to be able to give at this time is to stay up and wait. The battle is yours. Thank you for your promise to care for my children.

III

What Others See

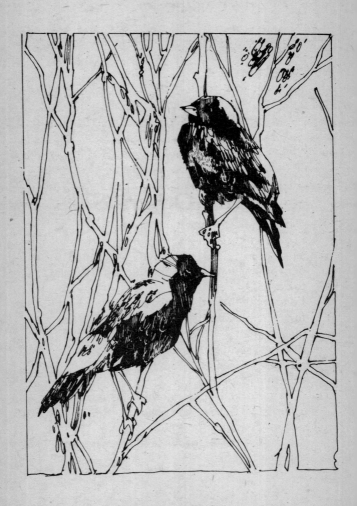

SMILE

Isn't there anyone who can smile at me, Lord?
  I want to tell them why we are dirty and why
  my baby is crying.
  They just look at me in disgust.
  I can almost hear them say,
    "Why do some people have children
    anyway?"
When I went to the coffee shop for a fresh
  bottle of milk to feed our baby, the waitress
  insisted that I pay first.
  Did she have to scald the bottle like it had
  never been washed before?
  Did she have to treat me so rudely?
Oh Lord, if only someone would show some
  sign of caring. I'd tell them that we rolled
  our car in Death Valley and that we are lucky
  to be alive.
  I'd also tell them that we are doing our best
  to get home. We know we are dirty. We are
  hungry, too.
  But most of all we are lonely for a smile.
May I learn one lesson from this dreadful
  experience.
  A smile costs the giver nothing but may open
  a world of hope for the receiver.
Teach me to smile.
  Teach me to care, to love, and teach me not
  to judge others.

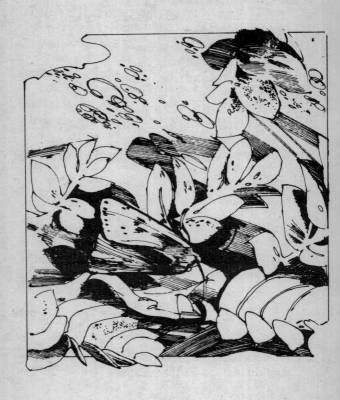

HONESTY HURTS

I am crying to you, Father, for help this day. I have come too far to go down in defeat now. You know the way that I bristle when she walks into the room. Her very presence causes me to put up my defenses. My actions yesterday were unkind and hurtful. The enemy tries to convince me that at least I was honest—and I was. But my honesty needed a sprinkle of gentleness and a cupful of love.

Hear my plea, O Lord. I do not have a love for her. I cannot in my own strength develop an ability to even like her, let alone love her. You see I need a miracle . . . a big miracle. Have mercy on me and fill me with gentleness and kindness. But most of all, fill me with a genuine love.

Right now I'll send her a note telling her that I would like to talk to her. When we meet may your love shine through me—let it be genuine—and may she see Jesus.

Grant me this favor. Rescue me and I will let the life of your love flow through me.

Cleanse me of self, chip off my stubbornness, and polish this relationship until it sparkles with patience, understanding and love.

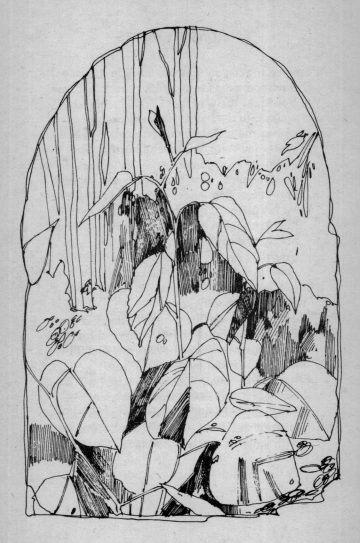

SEEKING FORGIVENESS

Lord Jesus, let me take a minute to thank you
for the events of this day. Truly, you have
blessed me beyond all measure.
I told her that I had not been gentle and that
I had been unkind. I told her that I was truly
sorry, and I asked her forgiveness. I couldn't
believe it when the tears came to her eyes—
when she held me close and said,
"Oh, thank you . . . it is a real pleasure to
meet someone who stands above the
crowd."
O God, may I soon be able to tell her that it is
you. It is you who stands above. I am
nothing. It is you. Blessed be the Lord who
makes my seemingly crooked way straight. I
will praise you all the days that I live.
Lead me each step that I may hear your
faintest whisper and feel your most gentle
nudge. Give me the courage to always admit
my faults and to ask forgiveness of those I
have wronged. May my honesty open many
doors for sharing your love with those in my
world.

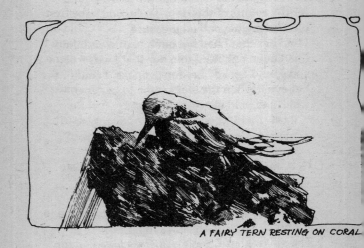

A FAIRY TERN RESTING ON CORAL

TOO COMMITTED

Dear Lord, free me from the conflicting commitments that I have at this hour. I am torn because of overcommitment.
When I promised that I would fulfill the first appointment, I was confident that I could do it. Now a more urgent need has arisen, and I am supposed to be in two places at the same time.

You are not the author of confusion. You have not planned for me to be uncertain of my direction. I plead with you to free my spirit, so that I can minister freely to this one in need.

Remove from me the selfish desire to satisfy my own nature. Give me confidence to honestly remove myself from my commitment to pleasure, and motivate me to humbly go and serve.

Thank you, Lord, for hearing my plea and for restoring my peace and stability. Grant me love and understanding from the one to whom I first said yes.

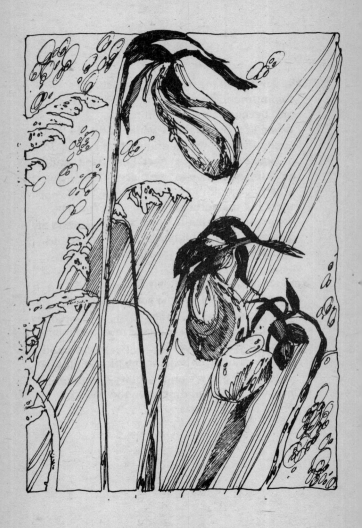

AVOIDANCE

Lord, when I see my friend's husband, I avoid
him. There is something about his manner
that says to me. "I don't accept you. I do not
have confidence in you."
He seems to have a subtle way of laughing at
me. That's why I walked all the way around
the building to keep from speaking to him
today.
Is there anyone to whom I give similar
vibrations? Do I make them feel foolish?
Please grant me the ability to make everyone
feel worthwhile and needed.
Give me confidence so that I will not feel small
when I am in his company. But may I always
remember this feeling, so I will be aware of
how I make others feel in my presence.

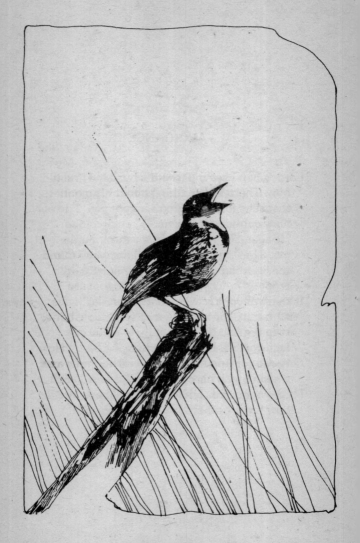

HARSH WORDS

Lord, I need an extra portion of love today. She
was so harsh with me over the phone. My
boys are playing basketball again. I find it
difficult to believe that the bouncing ball
bothers her that much.
"Send them to the school," she scolded.
"That's where mine played."
I wonder if that is why she is alone now. Could
it be the reason why they don't visit her?
What do I do now with the rolls that are
baking? I made them just for her. Will she
slam the door in my face? Perhaps I'd better
keep them.
"No, my child, I asked you to make them. Now
obey me. Ring her doorbell with a smile and
a wish for a blessed day."
Thank you, Lord. Thank you for always
knowing.

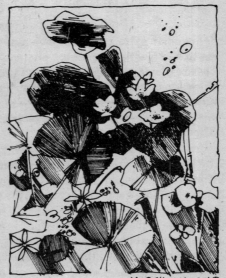

MARSH MARIGOLD

I HATE GOOD-BYES

Lord,
     It's Hard!
     Please Help!
     Give me confidence!
     I want to run. I don't want to tell anyone
     good-bye.
     I hate good-byes.
     Please let me disappear . . . become
     invisible . . . anything.
     I hate today.
     I don't like meaningless little words.
     There is nothing more to say. It is over.
     Why prolong the agony of departure?
I think I shouldn't get involved with people. I
need to keep to myself—fight my own battles—
and climb mountains alone—just quietly go my
way.

     I must guard myself and not let anyone
     near. No one should know. I'll wear a
     mask until I can leave this place today. I'll
     smile and be polite. I must not let myself
     feel. I will be strong.
I'll go my way. I won't let anyone near—no
one! If I am very still—like a tree—they won't
know. They will just walk by and not notice.

Jesus, what would you do?

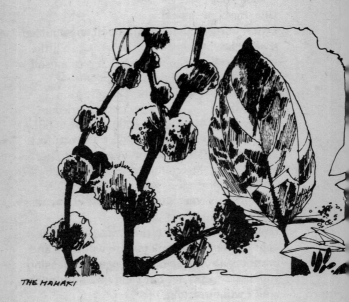

THE MAMAKI

ENVY

Lord, my problem today is envy. It is disguised
well. You see she always has things a little
bit better than I do. I try to convince myself
that it doesn't matter.

Help me. Free me from this tempting sin. I
desire to sing your praises this day. Your
nearness will keep me in line. Help me tell
everyone of your gracious words of comfort.
Let me show love in my every action to her.
Remind me that you have special blessings
for each of us.

Don't let this problem cripple my effectiveness
and my ministry for you.

Thank you for removing the anguish of envy
that I have felt. Thank you for who I am and
for the many ways in which you are blessing
my life. Thank you that I can now admire her
material gain and not feel inferior.

I praise your name.

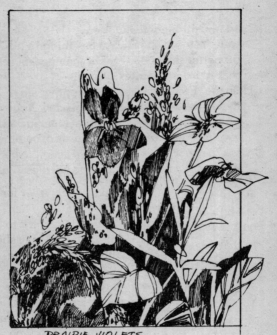

PRAIRIE VIOLETS

I CARE

Jesus, I know just where she is . . . where she
is living and serving. It is a time of giving
until it seems that to speak another word will
cause total collapse. Teach her the way of
renewal. Show to her how you went away so
often to pray alone, and how dependent you
were upon your Father. You had no one else
to guide you. No one human friend really
understood your ministry.

So it is with her. She is left to draw her only
strength and inspiration from the Father —
God. It seems that the demands are
overwhelming. But you had your priorities
set while you walked this earth. Teach her,
likewise, to tend to her own soul and to
nourish her own body and spirit in order for
her ministry to be without strain. May her
love flow freely from her confident spirit to
those who are in need this day. And may she
realize that it is the quality of time, not the
quantity that matters.

As she rests at your feet this day, show her
the simple amidst the seemingly complex.

I will praise your name throughout this day, for
you have heard my cry. You will set her on
her feet to touch lives with your seasoning.
Just a pinch is usually enough to make her
world tolerable.

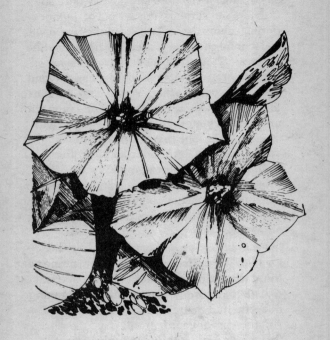

INSECURE

Lord, she appears to be shallow and trite. She
smiles freely enough and her words are
chosen with care. But her eyes look beyond
me in search of someone more impressive to
talk with. She controls our conversation with
framed questions. She is preoccupied with
her looks—adjusting her rings and
straightening her scarf.

Her insecurities are apparent and I desire to
help her. Why is it that I can't get her
attention? Why do we stand here and deal in
empty words when meaningful exchange is
available.

There she goes—a lonely person. I tried. I
failed. I pray that next time she'll let me near
and I'll be able to meet her where she is.

Be with her, Lord, and may she find meaning
and the freedom to be real.

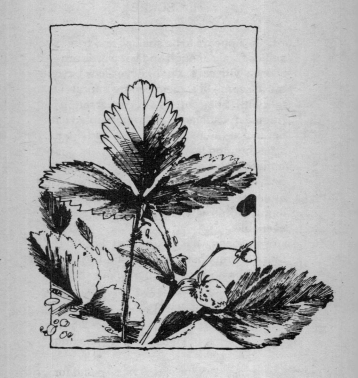

THE GIFT OF FRIENDSHIP

Lord Jesus, I want to thank you this day for
friends. Friends who understand how
desperately I need to get away from the daily
grind. Friends who have offered me the key
to their summer home.

And so here we are. You and I. We have this
quiet lakeside cabin to ourselves. For three
days no one will say, "Hey mom, what's for
dinner?" "Will you drop me by the school?"
"You're wanted on the phone." "Did you
mail my letters?"

I love my home and I love my family, but
sometimes they do not see beyond their own
immediate needs. I am always staying one
step ahead of them to see that they are
plugged into the right circuit at the right
time. I see that one is finished in the
bathroom before the next one needs it. I see
that his alarm doesn't wake her up. I make
sure he hasn't left all of his own lawn jobs for
one day. There's an endless list of "making
sure."

Thank you, Lord, for the gift of friends and for
their gift to me of these three quiet days.

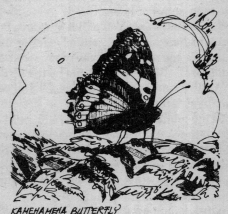

KAMEHAMEHA BUTTERFLY

MAKE ME WILLING

Lord, when he came to repair the sofa, I
    wanted him to get his job completed quickly
    and be on his way. It was an evening that I
    had set aside to be alone. I resented even
    this slight intrusion. By the time we had
    revised the federal government, and the
    local school district, I was falling completely
    apart and nearly pushing him out of my door.
Thank you for just the right words.
    ''Mr. Carlson, I will never be able to
    understand Watergate, and I am only one
    small part of this school district. I believe
    that change must start at the bottom—with
    you and me. Perhaps peace can only saturate
    the structure of our society one person at a
    time. Since the day that I accepted the fact
    that Jesus Christ really loves me, I have had
    peace. My individual world is in order . . . is
    yours?''
Lord, you knew that was to be the real
    beginning of our conversation. The trivia had
    been turned into meaning and purpose. We
    had passed over the symptoms and arrived
    at the source.
Thank you for allowing me the privilege of
    sharing your peace that evening, and for the
    opportunity of praying with Mr. Carlson.
    You knew all along that, one week later, he

would leave his earthly cares to be with you forever.

I pray that you will keep me sensitive to the needs of others. Open my eyes to the meaning behind idle conversation. Give me the courage to share my purpose for living. I may be the best Christian that someone else will ever know.

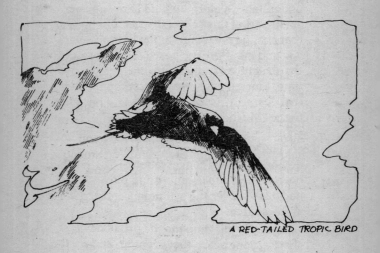

A RED-TAILED TROPIC BIRD

YOU AND I, LORD

It was you and I, Lord, when we began this
 spiritual pact. You reached out to me, and I
 reached back to you.
 We began our partnership that day. We
 agreed that you would make the decisions
 and I would co-sign.
 I would carry out the transactions, and you
 would provide the resources.
After the first agreement others were added to
 our partnership, and we became a small
 business. You still initiated the transactions
 and provided the resources, while I agreed to
 do your work.
How well I remember when you suggested that
 we incorporate and add new dimensions,
 new people, and new responsibilities. I
 found the agreement difficult to sign. But
 after much thought, I added my name.
Today our entire venture seems to be going
 bankrupt, and people are grumbling among
 themselves, causing unrest and friction.
Lord, I just want to remind you that I have let
 you control all. I have depended upon you
 and if, in the end, it is just the two of us—I
 haven't changed my mind.
We are partners—you and I.

OTHER GOOD BOOKS FROM HARVEST HOUSE